The Eyes  Have It

ALSO BY SUSAN REX RYAN

Defend Your Life II
Silent Inheritance
Defend Your Life

The Eyes Have It

A Patient's Insights Into Cataract Surgery

Susan Rex Ryan

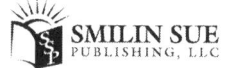

Copyright ©2020 by Susan Rex Ryan

All rights reserved.

No part of this book may be reproduced, stored in a retrieval system, or transmitted in any form or by any means, photocopied, electronically, mechanically, or otherwise, without prior permission by the copyright holder or publisher.

DISCLAIMER

The purchaser or reader of this book hereby acknowledges receiving notice of this DISCLAIMER. The author and SMILIN SUE PUBLISHING, LLC, publisher of this book, are not engaged in providing optical or medical care or services, and the information presented in this book is in no way intended as optical or medical advice or as a substitute for professional counseling. The information in this book is not intended to diagnose or treat any optical, medical or physical condition or problem. If optical, medical, professional, or other expert assistance is needed or required by the reader of this book, please seek the services of a competent expert. This book is based upon information taken from sources believed to be reliable. Although reasonable caution has been taken in compiling the information contained herein, this book may not contain the best or latest information and, in fact, may contain mistakes. The reader should use this book only as a general guide. The opinions expressed in this book are not to be relied upon as statements of fact. Anyone who reads or purchases this book, or any vitamin, mineral, or supplement mentioned in this book, acknowledge that they are relying upon their own investigation and not on any statements or opinions expressed herein, and are making their own independent decisions after discussions with their doctor or other medical professional. This book is sold without representation or warranty of any kind, express or implied, and the author and SMILIN SUE PUBLISHING, LLC are not liable or responsible to any person or entity for direct or indirect loss, damage, or injury caused or allegedly caused by information contained in this book.

Published in September 2020 by Smilin Sue Publishing, LLC.

smilinsuepubs.com

ISBN Print: 978-0-9845720-5-2
ISBN eBook: 978-0-9845720-6-9

Book design by BookWise Design.
Cover illustration by Celia Maria Ribeiro Ascenso.

Dedication

To my wonderful husband David.
You are my world.

CONTENTS

Introduction   1

THE GOOD

1. So, You Have Cataracts   5
2. Accepting the Need for Cataract Surgery   11
3. Preparing for Cataract Surgery   17
4. Imminent Preparations for Cataract Surgery   29
5. The Day of Surgery   33
6. Recovering from Cataract Surgery   39

THE BAD

7. The Eyeglasses Challenge   49
8. Pre-Existing Eye Issues   55
9. Short-Term Complications   61

THE UGLY

10. Diabetes Eye Complications   67
11. Dysphotopsia   73
12. Macular Degeneration   77
13. Post-Surgery Complications   81

Concluding Thoughts   89
Bonus Chapter: Eye Nutrition   91
Index   99
Glossary   103
Bibliography   111
Acknowledgments   115
About the Author   117

INTRODUCTION

The Eyes Have It is the book that I would have appreciated reading before my cataract surgeries. Yes, a book that candidly shares the experiences of a layperson going through the cataract surgery process.

Fortunately, my cataract surgeries were successes. My intermediate and far distances improved from lousy to 20/20. My new visual acuity has heightened to amazing detail and colors that burst with life. The outcome of my cataract surgery is a great gift!

To present a candid perspective, however, I divided *The Eyes Have It* into three parts. In addition, I included a bonus chapter on eye nutrition: tips for how to have healthier eyes before and after surgery.

The first part of *The Eyes Have It* is called "The Good" where I explain my experiences as a cataract newbie and add substantive discussion to the process.

While no one wants complications in cataract surgery, the truth is that it does happen. Statistics about the number and outcome of cataract surgeries vary from source to source. Suffice to say, approximately ten million cataract operations are performed annually worldwide, according to a variety of sources. About ninety percent of these surgeries are characterized as successful.

But what about the one million or so people who endure complications from cataract surgery? This is where the "The Bad" and "The Ugly" parts of this book come into play.

The second part of *The Eyes Have It*, referred to as "The Bad," addresses cataract surgery issues that can be resolved or treated. These complications range from dealing with new eyeglasses to short-term complications and pre-existing health issues.

The last part of the major body of the book is called "The Ugly" for obvious reasons. Yes, it is possible to have healthy eyes before surgery and end up with a surgery that degrades or ruins eyesight.

While there are no guarantees with the outcome of cataract surgery, I also include tips to improve the outcome of your surgery.

I sincerely hope that reading *The Eyes Have It* will prepare you for a positive outcome that may improve your quality of life. Best wishes,

—Susan Rex Ryan

THE GOOD

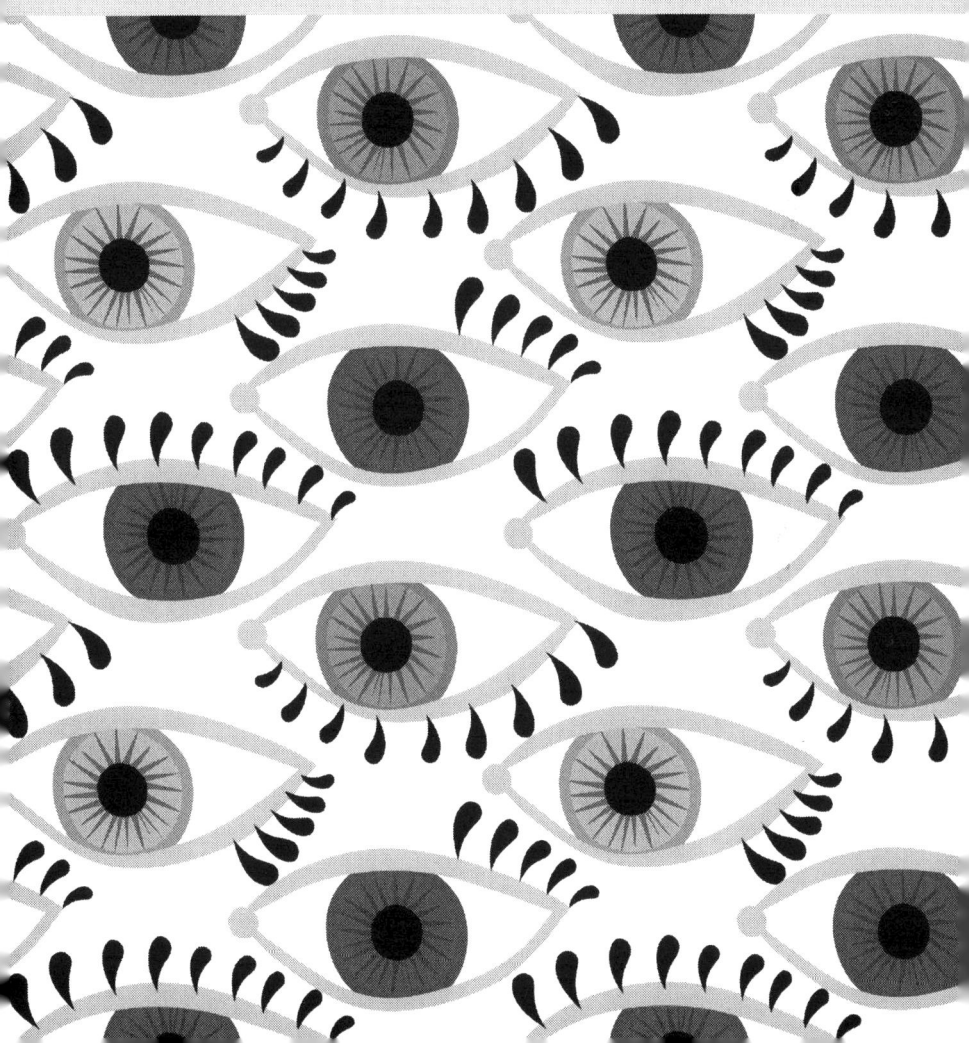

1

SO, YOU HAVE CATARACTS

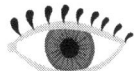

Going to the eye doctor and wearing glasses have been an integral part of my life since I was about 12 years old. Every year my mother faithfully shepherded me to crowded waiting rooms resplendent with adult eye patients, some wearing formidable-looking, dark glasses. These somewhat imposing visits continued during my undergraduate university years. Understanding the importance of healthy eyes, I continued the annual exams as an adult.

During an annual eye checkup when I was about 55 years old, my ophthalmologist commented that a cataract was beginning to form in my right eye.

"A cataract??? Isn't this an old person's eye condition?" I thought with some immediate dread.

"My maternal grandmother, mother, and father had cataracts. Oh, no! Not *me*..."

I recall inquiring how long before the cataract would become a vision issue. My ophthalmologist pointed out that each person is different. He told me that *I would tell him* when the cataract was beginning to impair my vision.

Within a year or so, the good doctor remarked that another cataract was developing, albeit slower than the first one, in my left eye.

For at least seven years since the first cataract was diagnosed, I did not notice any vision impairment except for annual but minimal changes in my eye prescription that I attributed to aging. However, during each annual examination, the doctor drew an image in my medical folder of the ever-growing cataract in my right eye. It was only a matter of time before I would hear two of the most dreaded words in my vocabulary: cataract surgery.

Discussion: Cataract Basics

Most people have heard of cataracts and understand that they are associated with the eyes. But *what is a cataract?* Simply stated, a cataract is the clouding of the natural eye lens.

Since ancient times, the word "cataract" has been identified in both the Greek and Latin languages as a "waterfall." An advanced cataract left untreated can resemble an image of cascading water and may lead to blindness.

Cataracts are a significant cause of visual impairment and blindness worldwide. The statistics are somewhat daunting. The World Health Organization estimates that more than 100 million natural eye lenses globally have a cataract.

More than twenty-four million Americans ages 40 and older have at least one cataract. By age 75, about half of all Americans have cataracts.

Understanding Cataracts

To understand cataracts is to first look at the natural eye lens, which helps focus light on the retina. (The light-colored surface in the back of the eye is the retina.) The natural eye lens comprises primarily water and protective proteins, called *alpha-crystallins*. Normal scattering of these proteins allows light to pass through the lens and focus images on the retina.

As we age, the alpha-crystallins proteins often clump together by a biological process called protein aggregation. The clumping accumulation of these proteins in the natural eye lens, hence, the cataract, blocks light and causes vision impairment. The only known cure for cataracts is surgical removal and replacement of the clouded, natural eye lens. Details about cataract surgery are discussed in Chapters 3 through 6.

Symptoms of cataracts are associated with vision degradation. These symptoms include blurry or cloudy eyesight; poor night vision; colors that appear to be faded; light issues such as halos, glare, and excess brightness; and frequent changes to eye prescriptions.

Types of Cataracts

Most cataracts are associated with aging. There are three classifications of age-related cataracts: nuclear, cortical, and subcapsular.

A *nuclear cataract* is the most common of age-related cataracts. The haze primarily in the center of the lens may indicate a nuclear cataract.

Cortical cataracts form along the edge of the lens. A shape that resembles the spokes in a bicycle wheel is indicative of a cortical cataract. Cortical cataracts are especially an issue for diabetic patients.

Subcapsular cataracts start at the front or back of the lens. This type of cataract tends to develop quickly.

A non-aging type of cataract is called *congenital* when a baby is born with, or develops, cataracts. *Traumatic* cataracts are the result of an eye injury, either recent or many years ago.

Risk Factors of Cataracts

Age is the greatest risk factor related to cataract development. Genetics also play a role in cataract development. In my case, I am aware of at least three generations in my family having cataracts.

Lifestyle choices, including smoking, unhealthy diet, excessive sunlight exposure, and taking steroid medications, are suspected as risk factors for the development of cataracts. The research community however has yet to prove that any of these lifestyle factors are causative. A way to prevent cataracts is to do the opposite of the high-risk lifestyle choices.

2

ACCEPTING THE NEED FOR CATARACT SURGERY

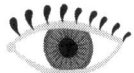

My ophthalmologist told me, plain and simple, that I will need cataract surgery in both eyes within a year or so. The mere thought of anyone cutting into my eyes was completely anathema to me. I really could not even think about the surgery, let alone face it. What on earth do I do?

Meanwhile, my ophthalmologist reassured me that he had performed thousands of successful cataract surgeries. He emphasized that all his surgeries were done without a hitch.

I could not help but think of my poor mother who had endured a botched-up surgery in her left eye. She does not remember however any details about what went wrong during the procedure. Suffice to say, since the surgery my mom has dealt with unresolved eye issues for decades. I do know that her retina was damaged during cataract surgery. Moreover, her sight in the affected eye is far from 20/20.

Cataract surgery is deemed safe and effective by the professional medical community. About three million Americans undergo cataract surgery each year. More than 98 percent of these procedures are deemed successful, according to the VisionAware™ organization. What about the poor two percent of Americans who have cataract surgery with complications? After all, two percent of three million persons comprise approximately 60,000 individuals who are diagnosed with adverse outcomes. That is a lot of failed procedures that affect a precious gift from birth: our eyesight!

Subsequently, I gave the idea of having cataract surgery a lot of thought and consideration. A summary of my research of the literature can be found in the below-mentioned "Discussion" section of this chapter.

In 2019, my ophthalmologist once again emphasized the absolute need for cataract surgery. Not only was my vision slowly deteriorating, but my driver's license was expiring. My age and state of residence required passing the eye test to issue an updated identification card. The necessity of having a valid driver's license cannot be understated. After all, this government-issued identification is required for everyday life, from credit card purchases to air travel. So, imminent renewal of the driver's license was the clincher! I had to make room in my busy schedule to accommodate the seemingly myriad eye appointments related to cataract surgery.

Discussion: Improving the Odds of Successful Cataract Surgery

Two major factors usually dictate the success of cataract surgery: the surgeon and place of surgery. One thing for sure is that you want your results to be in the top ninety percent of cataract procedures. Avoid being one of the ten percent of persons who enter surgery with healthy eyes and leave with a serious eye complication including possible blindness. Let's first look at the surgeon.

Eye surgeons are ophthalmologists by education, training, and skill. If you are seeing an optometrist, please understand that he or she cannot perform cataract surgery. Trusted optometrists however can be a good source for recommendations of ophthalmologists who perform cataract surgery.

Treat referrals from family and friends with caution because one or two successful surgeries with positive outcomes do not guarantee that you also will have flawless results. Try to find out the surgeon's track record. For example, my cataract surgeon <u>only performs cataract surgeries</u> and boasts over 9,000 successful procedures.

Another way to investigate potential eye surgeons is to do *due diligence* before selecting an eye surgeon for cataract removal and replacement. Contact your state boards of ophthalmology, optometry, and/or medical examiners. These organizations can tell you if a complaint has been filed against an ophthalmologist you are considering.

Pre-existing health conditions may increase your risk of surgery complications. These medical issues include glaucoma, diabetes, tobacco smoking, and high blood pressure. If you are an at-risk cataract patient, ensure that your eye surgeon is positively experienced in dealing with such complex issues.

Let's not forget the surgery setting. Cataract surgery is typically performed on an out-patient basis at a location separate from the office but is directly affected by the quality of the staff, equipment, and state of hygiene.

The nursing staff monitors your vital signs and diligently administers eye drops. The quality of the surgery equipment also is important. Does the surgery center have state-of-the-art, laser equipment for cataract surgery? Finally, check out the reviews and records of the surgery center regarding cleanliness and infection statistics.

3

PREPARING FOR CATARACT SURGERY

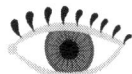

Be prepared to undergo a number (seven for me) of eye doctor appointments directly connected to your cataract surgery. I cleared my calendar for the month of the two cataract surgeries as well as several weeks prior to, and after, the operations. The more you understand about pre-surgery preparations beforehand, the better you should feel about the process.

The Initial Visit

About one month prior to my first scheduled surgery, I underwent the initial visit that entails examining the health of my eyes as well as obtaining physical eye measurements. After dilating my eyes, my ophthalmologist assessed them to ascertain if they were sufficiently healthy to undergo cataract surgery. Once the excellent health of my eyes was confirmed, a technician, using a couple machines in the office, measured the detailed physical aspects of each eye such as the curve of the cornea as well as the size and shape. (I was surprised to learn that one eye is larger than the other!)

The Pre-Op Appointments

Several days prior to each surgery, I had my pre-op appointment with an eye technician in the ophthalmologist's office. The eye technician proffered a low-key approach to the visit. She played a short video that clearly depicted the difference in vision distances between the monofocal intraocular lens (IOL) and the multifocal IOL.

She also asked me to read and sign a plethora of written acknowledgments and waivers about IOL and surgery selections that required my decisions and signature during this visit. I considered several factors before I made a final decision, including monetary costs, chances of success as well as astigmatism and presbyopia management.

Monetary Costs

Surprisingly, many patients of cataract surgeries incur thousands of dollars in costs. Costs depend on lens and surgical procedure selections. For example, the out-of-pocket costs for the *monofocal* IOL (strong probability to see either near or far distances but not both unless if you opt for *mini-mono vision*) laser-assisted procedure were $1,850 per eye plus healthcare insurance co-payments for the eye drops, ophthalmology surgeon, anesthesiologist, and surgery center. However, the procedure involving a *multifocal* lens (possibility of both near and distance visions) with laser surgery would be at least an additional $900 per eye out-of-pocket cost in addition to the co-payments associated with the surgery.

Please be advised that Medicare and private healthcare insurance plans only will cover the basic or traditional manual scalpel surgery (no laser-assisted) and a monofocal lens per eye. The mere thought of my eye being cut open by a scalpel was enough to freak me out! Fortunately, at least in the United States, most patients can opt to have a laser machine (called the femtosecond (FS) laser) make high-precision cuts instead of surgeon-handheld medical tools. (Please refer to the Discussions section of this chapter for additional information about lens and surgery options.)

Odds of Success

Based on information provided as well as my own *due diligence*, I believed that the odds of a successful outcome for the monofocal IOL procedure using laser surgery were higher than the mini-mono vision or multifocal IOL surgery using a FS laser. Why? The office indicated that some patients have serious issues with the multifocal lens.

The notion of a laser incising my cornea was not exactly comforting but I believed that laser-assisted surgery was the safer and more accurate option. (Please see the Chapter 2 discussion of "Improving the Odds of Cataract Surgery" for pertinent information.)

Astigmatism Management

Initially, I did not care about astigmatism management because I thought that I did not have this common condition. But the technician assured me that I do indeed have a slight astigmatism and pointed to the astigmatism data (a low cylinder power of 0.25 diopters) on my eye glass prescription.

Having an astigmatism indicated that I should opt for laser surgery. During cataract surgery the surgeon would make a tiny cut in the cornea (a "limbal relaxing incision") using the laser. Thus, the shape of the eye is corrected from an elongated (like an American football) form to a normal round shape (like a baseball).

Presbyopia Management

Presbyopia is a common condition in aging persons that makes it difficult for the eye to focus on near-distance vision. A person with presbyopia tends to hold reading material at arm's length to see it more clearly.

Fortunately, I was not diagnosed with presbyopia. This condition however can be corrected during cataract surgery by implanting specific types of IOLs. (Please see the discussion section later in this chapter for further information.)

The Surgery and IOL Decisions

So, for my right eye, I selected (in writing) the monofocal IOL with laser-assisted surgery for distance vision, which is apparently the most common option chosen by my ophthalmologist's patients. The laser-assisted surgery also would correct my mild astigmatism. With the monofocal lens, I would still need to wear reading glasses, which I did not think what a big deal. (Boy was I wrong! Please see Chapter 7 for my resolution of this issue.)

Eye Drops

Last but certainly not least, the technician gave me a list of three prescription eye drops that she submitted to a local pharmacy. I however was surprised at the total co-payment of $125 for these tiny bottles. The pharmacist assured me that my healthcare coverage and other discounts had already been applied to the prescription costs. The bottom line is that the drops are a required expense, and you will need to refill these drops at least once.

On the day before surgery, the eye-drop regimen began with two of the three prescribed eye drops. My right eye took one drop of an antibiotic three times on this day. In addition, I took one drop of a prescribed NSAID (non-steroidal anti-inflammatory drug). Little did I realize at the time that these drops would become a daily part of my life for weeks.

As the pre-op visit was wrapping up, the technician reminded me that on surgery day I would receive a gift of amazing sight (distance vision, in my case). In the next chapter we continue my journey on the "The Day of Surgery."

Discussion: Deciding On Cataract Surgical and Lens Options

The process of selecting the surgical procedures and lenses for your eyes can be complex and confusing. Yet it is a super-important decision that you must make *prior to* your cataract surgery.

Cataract Surgical Options

I have done my best to present this information in an easy-to-understand approach. There are two types of cataract surgery: traditional and laser-assisted. Here are explanations about both types of surgeries to help make an informed decision in concert with your ophthalmologist.

Traditional Surgery

The older traditional surgery option first entails using a scalpel to cut up to a ten-millimeter incision in the cornea. The surgeon then breaks up and removes the old cataract lens. After inserting the new intraocular lens (IOL), the incision may be sutured.

    The cost of the traditional surgery option is covered by Medicare and private healthcare insurance with the *proviso* that no laser-assisted procedures are performed during the cataract surgery. If a patient needs astigmatism correction under traditional surgery, an eyeglass prescription would be used to manage it.

Laser-Assisted Surgery

Modern laser-assisted surgery can be used to make a small precise incision in the cornea so the old cataract can be removed and replaced by a new IOL. In addition, *refractive laser* surgery can be used to reshape the cornea to improve astigmatism. Refractive laser surgery is performed by making a "limbal relaxing incision" to reduce or obviate your astigmatism.

It is important to note that you must need either management of astigmatism or presbyopia to justify using laser-assisted surgery. If you do not select, or are not eligible for, laser-assisted surgery, your cataract procedure will be performed manually by the surgeon, and your astigmatism will not be reduced by surgery. (Please note that the refractive laser procedure risk is higher for patients who have undergone LASIK surgery. This issue is further addressed in Chapter 8.)

Lens and Eyeglasses Options

Eyeglasses may be needed for your vision after cataract surgery. Vision zones include near, intermediate, and distance. For example, the range of intermediate vision is 20 inches (50 cm) (2.0 diopters) to 40 inches (50 cm) (1.0 diopter). Many people are reportedly comfortable with a vision at 26 inches (66 cm) (1.5 diopters). However, allow your eye doctor to help you decide what is the best vision for you.

Before selecting your IOL, you must decide if you are willing to wear glasses—at least part of the time—for the remainder of your life. The type of selected IOL and the success of the surgery determine the glasses requirement. As my ophthalmology staff clearly explained, patients must accept, in writing, specific risks associated with undergoing cataract surgery. (Please see Chapter 8 on risks from pre-existing eye issues.)

Let's first understand a little about the IOLs that are implanted in the eye to replace the cataract-damaged, natural lens. Most IOLs are made from pliable, acrylic plastic that is biocompatible, i.e., not harmful to living tissue. The intraocular lens (IOL) is not a new technology.

Over seventy years ago British ophthalmologist Harold Ridley, M.D. invented the IOL. He based his innovation on findings that the Royal

Air Force fighter pilots' eyes did not reject acrylic plastic splinters from shattered cockpit windscreens during World War II. In fact, the splinters appeared to float in the eyes. This discovery led Dr. Ridley to invent the IOL. Subsequently, he achieved his first permanent IOL implant in 1950.

In 1952, medical staff at Philadelphia's renowned Wills Eye Hospital performed the first IOL surgery in the United States.

Several options regarding the types of IOL and eyeglasses in cataract surgery include:

1. The most common type of IOL is called a *monofocal* lens, providing you near or distance vision. Eyeglasses would be required to see with the opposite of the type of monofocal you selected. In other words, a monofocal IOL with distance vision would mean that glasses for near vision would be necessary.

2. Another option, called modified monovision, or *mini-mono*, is to have one near-vision monofocal IOL in one eye and one distance monofocal IOL in the other eye. This strategy assumes that the brain adapts to the differing foci so you can see both near and far distances at the same time without eyeglasses. However, you still may need to wear eyeglasses.

3. The *multifocal* IOL provides a visual range that may afford far, intermediate, and near vision. This newer-generation multifocal lens works similarly to progressive lenses in eyeglasses. The option to potentially see well at all distances may obviate the need to wear eyeglasses after surgery. Do the multifocal lenses sound too good to be true? At least for some people, they are. Common complaints from patients who have multifocal IOLs include experiencing haze, glare, headaches, as well as a "halo effect" in the darkness.

For all IOLs, there is an additional option called a *toric lens*. In a nutshell, toric lenses were invented to fix or lessen pronounced astigmatism (approximately greater than or equal to 1.0 diopters). These lenses are more expensive than standard monofocal IOLs. While your chances of seeing well in the far distance with toric lenses increases, you still might need to wear eyeglasses after surgery. Your vision range is not guaranteed. In addition, toric lenses may be used to correct presbyopia as well as astigmatism.

You have the basic information to help you select the type of surgery, lenses, and eyeglasses options. You may realize that regardless of your selections, you still may need at least reading eyeglasses, a potential issue that I address in Chapter 7.

v

4

IMMINENT PREPARATIONS FOR CATARACT SURGERY

The day before my first surgery I was scared to death, plain and simple. I was absolutely petrified. For decades, I had heard about cataract surgery and hoped that I never would have to undergo the procedure. However, now I was facing the fact that cataract surgery was only hours away.

The Day Prior to Cataract Surgery

Of course, there are a few procedures to follow the *day prior to cataract surgery*: eye drops, washing, and fasting.

As I mentioned in Chapter 3, I was prescribed three types of eye drops. Two of the three drops began on the day before the surgery. I administered the prescribed antibiotic eye drop three times. In addition, I took one dose of the prescribed NSAID eye drops. My ophthalmologist instructed me to allow about three-to-five minutes between drops. (Please note: the use and type of eye drops may vary by the ophthalmologist.)

The doctor advised bathing or showering the night before surgery as most cataract procedures require being at the surgery center early in the morning. This is a great idea as patients are typically required to limit bathing near the eye at least a week.

Like other surgical operations and procedures, fasting (all food and beverages) as of midnight was also instructed.

The Morning of Cataract Surgery

The doctor's directions for what to do, or not do, are generally common sense and typical of instructions on the day of any surgery.

On the morning of my surgery, I took my morning medications per my ophthalmologist's instructions. The doctor stated a couple exceptions: 1) do not take insulin (bring it with you to the surgery center) and 2) if you are asthmatic, bring your inhaler with you to surgery.

Another instruction was to not wear any cosmetics, cologne, or perfume during the morning of surgery. (Wait until you read about post-surgery instructions about wearing makeup!)

Patients who do not feel well prior to the surgery date should contact their surgeon for a probable rescheduling of the appointment. Anesthesiologists do not allow patients with colds, flu, and other illnesses in surgery because these temporary conditions may interfere with the delivery of oxygen to the body. (Thankfully, I was healthy.)

A totally common-sense instruction was to not bring any money or other valuables with you as well as not to wear any jewelry. I gave my payment and identification cards to my husband who drove me to and from the surgery center.

Speaking of being transported, patients were required to arrange a responsible party to drive you to and from the surgery center. Ride-sharing companies and taxis are usually not considered a "responsible party."

Chapter 5 describes my observations on the dreaded day of cataract surgery.

5

THE DAY OF SURGERY

The day of dread began in the wee hours of the morning. Way too early for me but today I felt numb due to sheer fear. This really isn't happening, is it?

My husband Dave, who drove me, and I entered a cold, medicinal, empty—save for one man—waiting room. We barely sat down when the receptionist called my name. She checked my photo identification and charged the insurance co-payment to my credit card. I handed the two cards to my husband for safe keeping as no valuables were allowed in a patient's possession during the procedure.

We momentarily sat down before a nurse called my name. I bade good-bye to Dave (we were told that family members could not enter the pre-op area) and slowly walked with a staff member into the preparation area.

The nurse led me to a dressing area where I changed into one of those ill-fitting cloth gowns. They weighed me on a gigantic, flat stainless-steel scale. The type I have seen for farm animals.

She also marked a big black "X" over my right eye to ensure that everyone knew what eye was undergoing surgery today.

A staffer led me to a hospital-type recliner in a small open area. I had company: two patients and surprise, their spouses and an adult daughter. Everyone looked at me, apparently thinking, "Ah, we have company."

A warm blanket was placed over my lower body. The warmth was soothing during a time when small comforts are greatly appreciated.

I shut my eyes, trying to ignore the awkward situation. Suddenly I sensed a nurse slowly sauntering by me. I peeked at her with one eye slightly open.

"I see you peeking at me!" cackled an older woman with unkempt short white hair. Meet my "Nurse Ratched."

Nurse Ratched began to administer seemingly endless rounds of dilation and numbing eye drops. She also took my order for a post-operation beverage: cranberry juice. And she snatched my eyeglasses. (I did not realize until after the first surgery that I would never wear them again.)

I was finally led to another waiting room, this time with one other patient, a man who appeared to be around my age. His eyes sparkled from the muddy, sun-aged face and framed by a handlebar mustache. He seemed relaxed and told me that he was in for his second cataract surgery. This gentleman raved over the first surgery and the results. A little comfort that perhaps things would not be too bad. After all, he was back after two weeks for another round.

Another person entered the small waiting area and introduced himself as my anesthesiologist. He gave a small IV dose of versed and fentanyl for mild sedation. (I did not feel any pain during the surgery.)

Soon my new buddy headed into surgery. I bade him good luck. Within a couple minutes, an older woman was brought in as my next "roommate." She looked frightened and hesitantly nodded to my "hello." A minute later a woman entered our cramped space to interpret for her mother. They spoke Bulgarian!

I was next to WALK into the operating room. As I left the hospital chair, I smiled at the other patient and bade her well in Russian. Her eyes lit up, and she smiled. (Having visited Bulgaria years ago, I recalled that Russian was a mandatory subject in school. I assumed she would understand Russian, and she did.) Our short discourse made me feel like myself and eased my nerves a bit.

The nurse led me into a cold, noisy operating room with two imposing machines. I greeted my eye surgeon who was seated at a laser machine, called the femtosecond (FS) laser.

A nurse carefully helped ease me onto a stretcher-like, examination seat, told me not to be nervous, and strapped me into the seat. Then she proceeded to hold my head in place with something like duct tape. I also vaguely recall the nurse placing a device near my eye called a *speculum* to prevent blinking. I was scared to death.

My surgeon told me to be very still and turned on the laser. Realizing that the laser was going to incise my cornea, I felt as if I would "freak out." I overheard the surgeon and anesthesiologist commenting on my heavy, deep breathing. Then I just held it together and watched what could be best described as a "fireworks show."

After my surgeon said that the laser-assisted surgery went well, I was led to the other machine and climbed on the seat. A rubber tent with a hole in it for the eye was lowered over my head. I do not remember much else.

My next recollection was sipping cranberry juice in the recovery room, wearing a plastic shield over my operated eye, and being led by my dear husband to our car. In complete sincerity I asked him, "Do you have my glasses?"

Discussion: Cataract Removal and Replacement

If you are interested in how my cataract was removed and replaced with a monofocal intraocular lens (IOL), this brief discussion is for you. It is worth repeating that I endured no uncomfortableness or pain during cataract surgery. I attribute this to the surgeon's amazing skill, effective eye drops, as well as precision surgical procedures and equipment.

My eye surgeon performed a cataract surgery procedure called *extracapsular cataract extraction*. Through a two-millimeter incision (cut using the FS laser beam), he removed the faulty natural lens (cataract) from its elastic capsule and inserted a new foldable IOL (with the appropriate eye prescription) into the capsule.

A newer technique for cataract surgery called *phacoemulsification* also was used during the extraction procedure. About 95 percent of cataract surgeries are performed using phacoemulsification. My eye surgeon inserted a vibrating ultrasound probe that directed sound waves into the cataract nestled inside the transparent membrane capsule. Using the probe's vacuum, the surgeon broke the hard core of the cataract into pieces and suctioned them from the capsule. Hence, the empty capsule was ready for the insertion of the new foldable monofocal IOL. The entire surgery procedure took about twenty minutes. *Voila!*

6

RECOVERING FROM CATARACT SURGERY

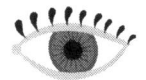

What a relief to know that my cataract surgery was over! Furthermore, my distance vision in my corrected eye was amazing. I regained a visual acuity that I only vaguely recollected from childhood. Not only was my far-distance eyesight incredibly clear but colors appeared to be more vibrant.

And I could see far distances well, including driving, *without* my glasses! In fact, my ophthalmologist gave me a wallet-size card for each eye with proof that I had cataract surgery in case law enforcement would question why I was driving without corrective lenses.

I soon realized that I would *never* again need to wear my pair of eyeglasses with expensive, tri-focal progressive lenses and a strong prescription. (The issue of eyeglasses after cataract surgery is addressed in Chapter 7.)

My operated eye felt fine except for mild itching. And I had to resist temptation to rub the eye because it is forbidden to do so.

The World of Eye Drops

Prescription eye drops rule after cataract surgery. In fact, my doctor advised starting the three types of drops in the operated eye immediately after surgery.

For the next week I took antibiotic drops three times a day, prednisone (steroidal) eye drops for every waking two hours, and non-steroidal anti-inflammatory drug (NSAID) eye drops once daily. According to my ophthalmologist, diligently following the eye drop course is key to successful recovery from cataract surgery.

Not only are there a lot of eye drops to be given each day but someone (the patient or home partner) needs to adequately put the drops in the eye. Furthermore, it is imperative that the person handling the eye drops washes his/her hands prior to administering the drops.

Many patients administer their own eye drops. In my case, my husband usually gave them to me. To attain the correct dosing, the eye drop administrator needs to closely focus the dropper on the center of the eye but without touching the eye. The patient needs to keep the operated eye wide open and stay focused on a spot on the ceiling until the drops are coolly felt on the eyeball.

Seven days after cataract surgery I underwent another post-operation appointment to learn that the eye drop regimen continued for 15 additional days! At least in my case, the eye drops were a bit less than the first week post-surgery. The prednisone eye drops were taken three times a day for five days, twice a day for another five days, and once daily for a final five days. As far as the NSAID drops are concerned, they are taken once a day until the bottle is empty. Oh, and it is important to wait five minutes between administering the next drop. You can see that eye drops do rule for almost a month after cataract surgery.

Post-Surgery Guidelines

As with any surgical procedure, there are activities that are encouraged or forbidden after the surgery. Of course, your eye surgeon's requirements should supersede those stated here within.

You Can:

- Eat regularly, watch TV, read, or take a walk.
- Wear sunglasses outside for at least a week after surgery.
- Blow your nose and cough *gently*.
- Wash your hair one day after surgery but avoid getting soap or water near the operated eye.
- Wear the plastic patch over your operated eye until the surgeon advises otherwise.

You Cannot:

- Drink any alcoholic beverages for the initial 24 hours after surgery.
- Get water into your operated eye for the first week after surgery. If you shower, keep your face away from the nozzle.
- Use swimming pools, hot tubs, or saunas for the first week, post-surgery.
- Wear eye cosmetics from 2–8 weeks, depending on your surgeon's instructions.
- Rub or touch your operated eye.
- Lift heavy objects or bend at the waist.
- Forget about your eye drop regimen! There may be overlap days when both operated eyes require the prescription eye drops.

Post-Operation Appointments

I had two post-operation appointments per operated eye. The first one was the day after surgery to check the health of the eye as well as vision performance. Eye pressure was fine. When I read the eye chart with my newly operated, the eye technician exclaimed, "Wow! 20/20 distance vision!" I was thrilled.

The second office visit occurred about six days after surgery. When the technician asked how my operated eye was doing, I replied, "OK. But I feel like something in my eye." The tech deadpanned, "Yes, it's a stitch. The doctor is going to remove it today!"

A stitch in my eye?!? No one even hinted at having a stitch but apparently for my ophthalmologist it is his normal procedure to suture the incision so his patients could avoid wearing a shield for a couple weeks. Fortunately, I had little time to be afraid of this action.

After getting numbing drops, I placed my chin on the *slit lamp*. With a pair of surgical scissors, the good doctor snipped the suture and pulled it slowly out of my eye. Although the procedure was a bit unnerving, it was quick and totally painless.

Two months after my initial cataract surgery I was required a follow-up appointment with my ophthalmologist. After examining the vision and health of both eyes, he proclaimed, "Perfect!"

Before we venture into "The Bad", I offer a brief discussion of the second surgery.

Discussion: The Second Eye Surgery

Normal cataract protocol includes removal of a cataract from each eye in two discreet surgeries. The second cataract operation usually occurs about two weeks after the first one. However, it is possible to undergo the second surgery within a week of the first surgery or more than two weeks after the first surgery. The decision is primarily the eye surgeon's.

The time between surgeries is certainly helpful in terms of the healing process. However, during the off time you most likely will notice an imbalance of vision between the two eyes. The brain tries to accommodate the vision capabilities of both eyes. Usually it is not a big deal but if you feel your vision needs balancing, avoid driving and using machinery until your second eye has its new IOL and is on the mend. Or you can remove the lens from one side of the eyeglasses to use until you undergo the second surgery.

My second cataract surgery went incredibly well. I think the main reason was that I had the experience of the first surgery behind me. Please do not get me wrong, I was still quite nervous during the morning of the second operation.

My second operated eye felt great after surgery. But I did have to have a stitch removed. I just sucked up the fear and did not feel a thing. A happy ending.

Some patients are not as fortunate to a happy ending. The part of the book called "The Bad" is next.

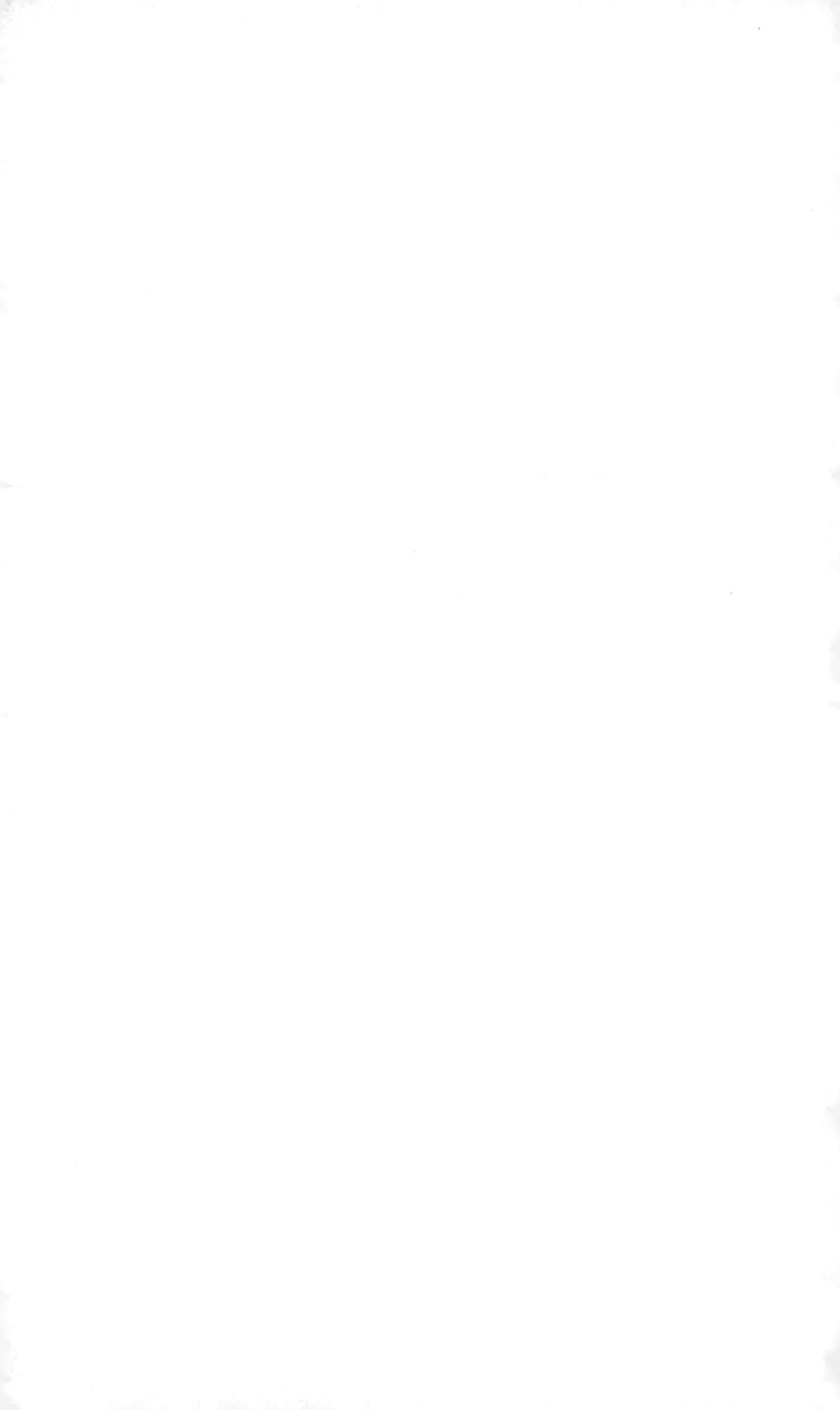

THE BAD

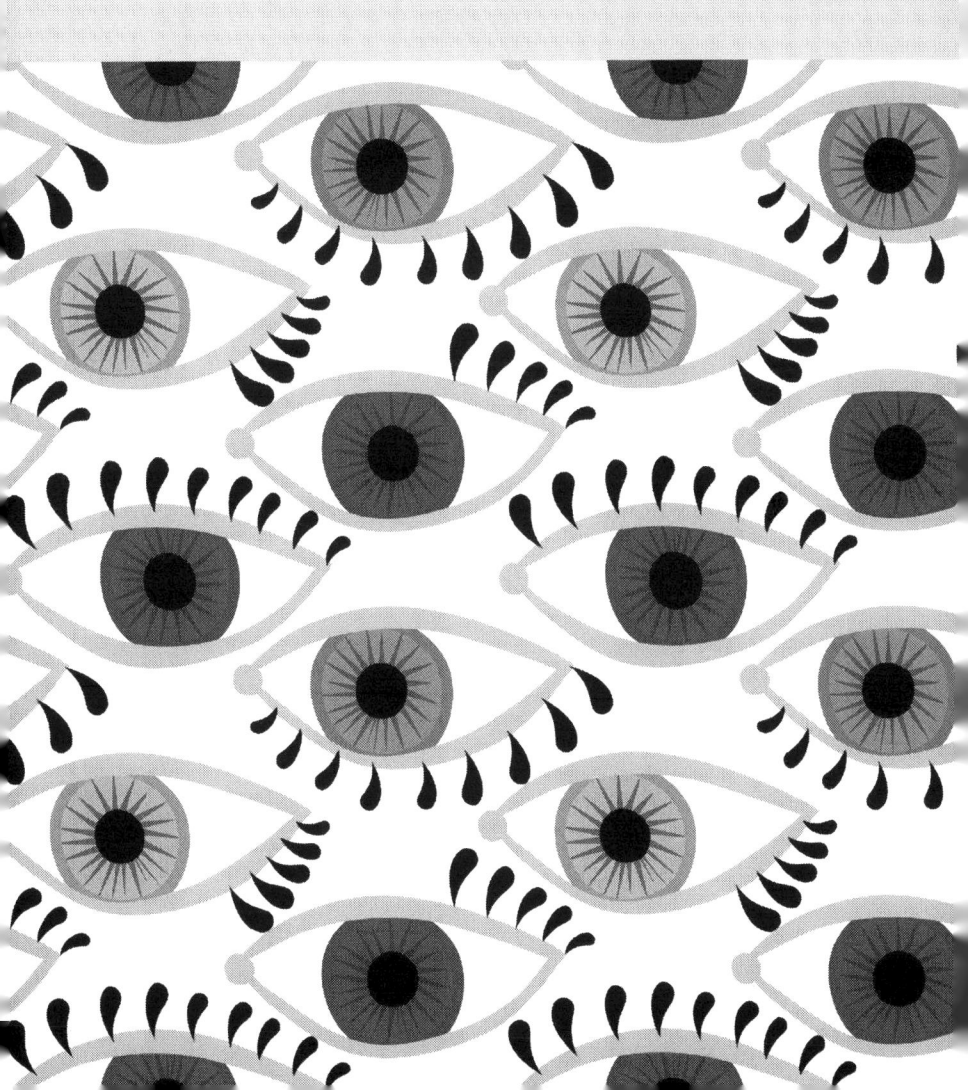

7

THE EYEGLASSES CHALLENGE

Eyeglasses are, at one time or another, a reality for almost everyone. I started wearing eyeglasses at the age of twelve years old. They fit right in as my image of a bookish nerd.

Four years later, looking ahead to college, I switched to hard contact lenses. (The technology of soft lenses was in its infancy.) But contact lenses were cumbersome to apply and wear. They would occasionally fall out of my eyes, for example. So, the eyeglasses went back on during my undergraduate years.

Wearing eyeglasses used to carry a variety of stigmas: intelligent, nerdish, mentally ill, and other perceptions of medical issues. But something changed; so many younger people are wearing eyeglasses these days that glasses have become a fashion accessory. Furthermore, for the older folks the propensity of wearing reading glasses allows for an inexpensive way of matching them to clothes or accessories. I do not think that wearing glasses has much of a stigma well in to the 21st century.

Presbyopia

Wearing eyeglasses was simply part of my landscape for decades. Except for the couple years of wearing contact lenses, I wore glasses for all distances every day of my life until I walked out of that surgery center after my first cataract operation. I knew that I would need readers after the second surgery but here's the "bad" thing…

My near vision prior to each cataract surgery was nearly perfect. Now it was not. The frustration to be unable to read anything up close without some type of lenses was greater than I had anticipated. Unfortunately, I quickly realized that—as the result of the far-distance, monofocal IOL that I selected for implantation—I had become presbyopic!

Presbyopia is a common eye condition that adversely affects near-vision in persons about 40 years or older. The condition occurs when the flexible muscles that hold the natural lens begin to stiffen with age. Cataract surgery literally disconnects those muscles from the natural lens.

No one emphasized the need for presbyopia-correcting lenses, probably owing to the price tag. The *additional* costs of non-toric, presbyopia-correcting IOLs—$1,800 for both eyes, and $3,200 for toric, presbyopia-correcting IOL in both eyes—exceeded my budget.

Furthermore, patients with presbyopia-correcting lenses frequently experience glare and halos around lights at night. In addition, blurry or foggy vison is quite common for both near- and far-distance visions, frequently attributed to refractive error. Ironically, eyeglasses (or contact lenses) were used for treatment!

The cruel reality set in that I would be stuck with presbyopia for life. At the time I thought I would just wear inexpensive "readers." Little did I know how annoying and an inconvenience readers were for me.

Reading Glasses

Readers, or reading glasses, are commonly used and widely available. I thought little about them until I went shopping for them after the second cataract surgery. Brick-and-mortar retail stores and pharmacies display readers on a rack crammed with other products. Alternatively, you can buy readers at online stores, but you cannot, of course, try them on for looks or readability.

    I initially shopped at a retail pharmacy for a style that I liked and looked at myself wearing them by peering into a small mirror atop the readers rack. Once I found a frame I liked, I searched for the right magnification—in this case, a +2.75 magnification where the print appears 2.75 times larger when wearing these glasses. Then I read the small print on product labels on nearby shelves to ascertain the lens' strength; I seemed to read fine with them (or so I thought). So, I selected a pair of reading glasses with a +2.75 magnification.

    After I was home from the store, I discovered two points of interest: first, I was reaching for the pair of readers almost constantly as I needed them to read anything on my phone or anything else. I also realized that a +2.75 magnification was too strong because a whopping headache would ensue, especially when I was reading on my laptop monitor.

    Long story short and a few different lens strengths later, I gradually went down to +1.50 magnifications and ended up having a pair of reading glasses in almost each room of the house! After reaching for a pair of glasses countless times a day, my patience ran out. (Due to the magnification of the lenses in reading glasses, you cannot wear them for intermediate and far distance vision owing to distorted sight.)

The solution to my constant frustration was not cheap but it worked well for me. I bought thin, titanium frames with progressive lenses made from clear glass for my 20/20 intermediate and far vision, while the lower part of the lenses was magnified +1.5.

My eyeglasses are so light and almost transparent that I look as if I am not wearing glasses! And more importantly, I do not have to take the glasses off and on scores of times per day! By the way, I priced non-progressive lenses (the lines in the lenses are prominent) for this concept. The cost was still over $400 for the lenses alone!

Before purchasing expensive eyeglasses, a mixture of luck afforded me an opportunity to check the accuracy of my +1.50 reading glasses in Phnom Penh, the capital city of Cambodia, of all places. My traveling companion lost her readers en route to Southeast Asia. Right across the street from our hotel was a modern optical shop!

An optician readily measured my friend's vision using a basic refractor. Within about twenty minutes, he produced a new pair of reading glasses for her.

While awaiting her new glasses, I asked the optician if he would measure my eyes for reading.

The refractor measured +1.50 for near distance. Therefore, I confirmed the correct reading strength prior to investing in these expensive permanent glasses in the United States!

Understanding that you most likely are not headed to Cambodia anytime soon, how can you get your correct magnification measured free-of-charge? One option is to visit an optician or an optometrist. Another alternative is to print one of the reading charts available for free on the Internet.

The bottom line is do due diligence of your lens and surgical options stated in Chapter 3. If I could do the surgery again, I would have made the same decision: laser-assisted surgery and monofocal IOL for intermediate and far distances vision. But I am perfectly content wearing almost "invisible" glasses. The decisions are yours to make.

In the next chapter I address how pre-existing medical conditions may adversely affect the outcome of cataract surgery.

8

PRE-EXISTING EYE ISSUES

You may recall in Chapter 3; I discussed the initial cataract examination to assess eye health and obtain critical eye measurements. Fortunately, my eyes were healthy and ready for cataract surgery. However, common eye conditions, including previous refractive surgery and glaucoma, may complicate cataract surgery.

Complicated Eyes

All eyes are not created equally. I was surprised when my ophthalmologist told me that my right eye is larger than the left. Who knew?

One common complication is called *small pupils*. The pupil is the surgeon's window into the eye; it must be open wide enough to perform safe cataract surgery. Despite using dilation eye drops, the pupil may not be large enough to allow the surgeon to perform cataract surgery. In today's world the surgeon can implement special intraocular devices to stretch temporarily and dilate the pupil. Eye surgeons also have methods to stabilize the iris.

Certain prescriptions drugs can affect the size of the pupil by weakening the iris. Ironically, a medication called pilocarpine, used to treat lower eye pressure, may permanently restrict the dimensions of the pupil. Some prescription drugs for high blood pressure, kidney stones, and urinary tract infections can adversely affect the size of the pupil. Therefore, it is imperative that you share the entire list of your medications at the initial examination.

The *capsular bag* holds the eye lens. The bag is suspended by *zonules*, thousands of microscopic fibers. Some people have a weakened capsular bag and/or zonules, making the operation more challenging and increasing the risk of complications during cataract surgery. This weakening may be caused by prior eye surgery, previous trauma, or retinopathy.

Pseudoexfoliation is another pre-existing complication. It is commonly known as "eye dandruff" and may cause damage to the iris muscles. Please see Chapter 12 for a detailed explanation of this "ugly" condition.

Glaucoma

Glaucoma is an "almost invisible" serious disease that gradually impairs peripheral vision. Normally, the eye constantly produces a clear fluid called *aqueous humor* that circulates inside the front part of the eye through a complex filtration system. When the drainage ducts become clogged or less efficient (more likely with age but even a baby can have glaucoma), the fluid builds up in the eye, causing intraocular pressure (IOP). If the IOP continues to rise, this pressure can cause gradual damage to the optical nerve. Treatment involves using various prescription eye drops and/or an operation called trabelculectomy, also called filtration surgery. The surgeon opens a new pathway, so the fluid bypasses the drainage system that is not working properly.

One common way to detect and track glaucoma is to measure IOP using a tonometry or "air puff" test. You simply place your chin on the brace of the tonometer, which is mounted on a slit lamp.

A puff of air quickly flattens the corneal surface, allowing the measurement of the eye's resistance to the puff.

A more accurate screening tool for glaucoma, however, is called the Goldmann applanation tonometry. Prior to this test, the technician administers numbing drops containing a yellow fluorescein dye, which glows under the tonometer's blue light. The doctor lightly presses the tip of a tiny probe to make an indentation on the cornea. The IOP is measured by the amount of force required to flatten the cornea.

If you have glaucoma, you can still have cataract surgery. In fact, some eye surgeons combine both a trabelculectomy and cataract surgery during the same appointment. However, research indicates that glaucoma outcomes may improve if they are dealt with prior to cataract surgery. On the other hand, cataract surgery sometimes offers a beneficial glaucoma result by lowering the pressure in the eye. It is important to note that reduced IOP varies from patient to patient. In fact, it is nearly impossible to predict the IOP outcome. Your ophthalmologist can weigh the possibilities with you.

LASIK

A popular eye procedure called LASIK (*laser-assisted in situ keratomileusis*) is a type of refractive surgery for the correction of nearsightedness, farsightedness, or astigmatism. LASIK is performed by an ophthalmologist who uses a laser to reshape the cornea to improve visual acuity.

Patients who have undergone LASIK can usually have cataract surgery. However, the ophthalmologist faces a challenge invoked by LASIK surgery, which reshapes the cornea. Thus, the measurement power of the modified cornea could be inexact. These potentially inaccurate dimensions would be used to calculate the power for the IOL that would replace the cataract lens.

However, if you have had LASIK surgery, you can help improve the likelihood that the power measurements of your LASIK-affected cornea are accurate. Providing your medical records of your pre- and post-operative data from the LASIK (or other previous refractive) surgery to your ophthalmologist is essential for a positive outcome. Remember that if the IOL power calculations are incorrect, your eye surgeon may have to increase the IOL strength or even implant an additional IOL on top of the first new lens.

Vitrectomy

It is not uncommon for people to have a vitrectomy prior to needing cataracts. A vitrectomy is outpatient surgery to treat issues with the retina and vitreous. The vitreous is a gel-like substance that fills about two-thirds of the volume of the eye. If floaters adversely affect vision, some people insist on a vitrectomy. This decision should be carefully considered. Why?

Patients who undergo a vitrectomy are highly likely (up to 100 percent) to need cataract surgery! A big downside to a vitrectomy is that a cataract usually begins to form not long after vitreous surgery. Yes, cataracts are common side effects of vitrectomies.

Let's say that there are many potential complications to performing cataract surgery on a patient who underwent a vitrectomy. Lots of extra care is required by the cataract eye surgeon to successfully perform cataract surgery. An example includes avoiding acrylic or multifocal IOLs.

In the next chapter we will discuss temporary complications *after* cataract surgery.

9

SHORT-TERM COMPLICATIONS

Short-term complications can occur after cataract surgery. They usually are obvious within a few hours to days after the cataract operation.

Bleeding

Bleeding in the eye can occur from cataract surgery. It is rare, though, because the incision normally is in the clear area of the cornea where there are no blood vessels. The iris, however, can bleed if it is accidently cut or nicked. If the iris is bleeding, the eye surgeon usually seals the bleeding spot by cauterization. (Please see information about Suprachoroidal Hemorrhage in the Ugly part of this book).

Dry Eye

Experiencing a condition called *dry eye* is not unusual after cataract surgery. Dry eye usually is a short-term annoyance. After even a minimal cataract incision is made, the eye surface is more comfortable when it is well lubricated. The solution to treating dry eye is to lubricate them with preservative-free artificial tears—in addition to your prescription eye drops. Preservative-free, artificial tear drops are readily available over the counter at retail supermarkets and drug stores.

Do not hesitate to tell your eye doctor about dry eye, despite its prevalence. Researchers from India concluded in a 2019 study that manual cataract surgery increases the risk of enduring dry eye. Phacoemulsification is the better option as the incidence of dry eye is improved due to laser-assisted precision rather than manual incision surgery.

Floaters

Floaters, clumps of vitreous gel in the central eye cavity, are commonly noticed after cataract surgery. It is important to note, though, that many people already have age-related floaters *prior to* cataract surgery. So, cataract patients often see pre-existing floaters after surgery when one's vision becomes so much clearer.

According to a study published in a 2018 issue of *the International Journal of Medical Sciences*, eye surgeons have the capability to release some ophthalmic viscoelastic devices (OVDs) used during the phacoemulsification (discussed in Chapter 5) phase of cataract surgery. By doing so, the likelihood of post-surgery floaters can be decreased.

Gritty Sensation

A common patient complaint is a gritty sensation in the operated eye. During cataract surgery the eyelids, of course, are open, causing the eyeball to dry. Despite a constant lubrication of the eyes with a special saline solution, dry spots still may occur. These spots eventually disappear. Meanwhile, quality lubrication eye drops, available over the counter, should help ease the gritty sensation.
As with all side effects, please be sure to tell your ophthalmologist about them.

Leaking Incision

The internal pressure in the eye naturally holds the cataract-related incision together so the cornea heals. However, when necessary, a tiny suture can be sewn to prevent leakage. Nonetheless, if the wound leaks, it could lead to serious infection including endophthalmitis (explained in Chapter 12).

Secondary Glaucoma

A condition called "secondary glaucoma" is an increase in eye pressure *after* cataract surgery. Although increased eye pressure post-surgery is unusual, it can cause symptoms ranging from nausea to blurriness and aching around the eye. The risk for secondary glaucoma is increased if your eye has bleeding or inflammation.

Fortunately, secondary glaucoma is usually temporary. Nonetheless, treatments include prescription eye drops and laser-assisted treatment to alleviate the fluid and decrease the eye pressure.

The next chapter of this book is referred to as "The Ugly" for obvious reasons.

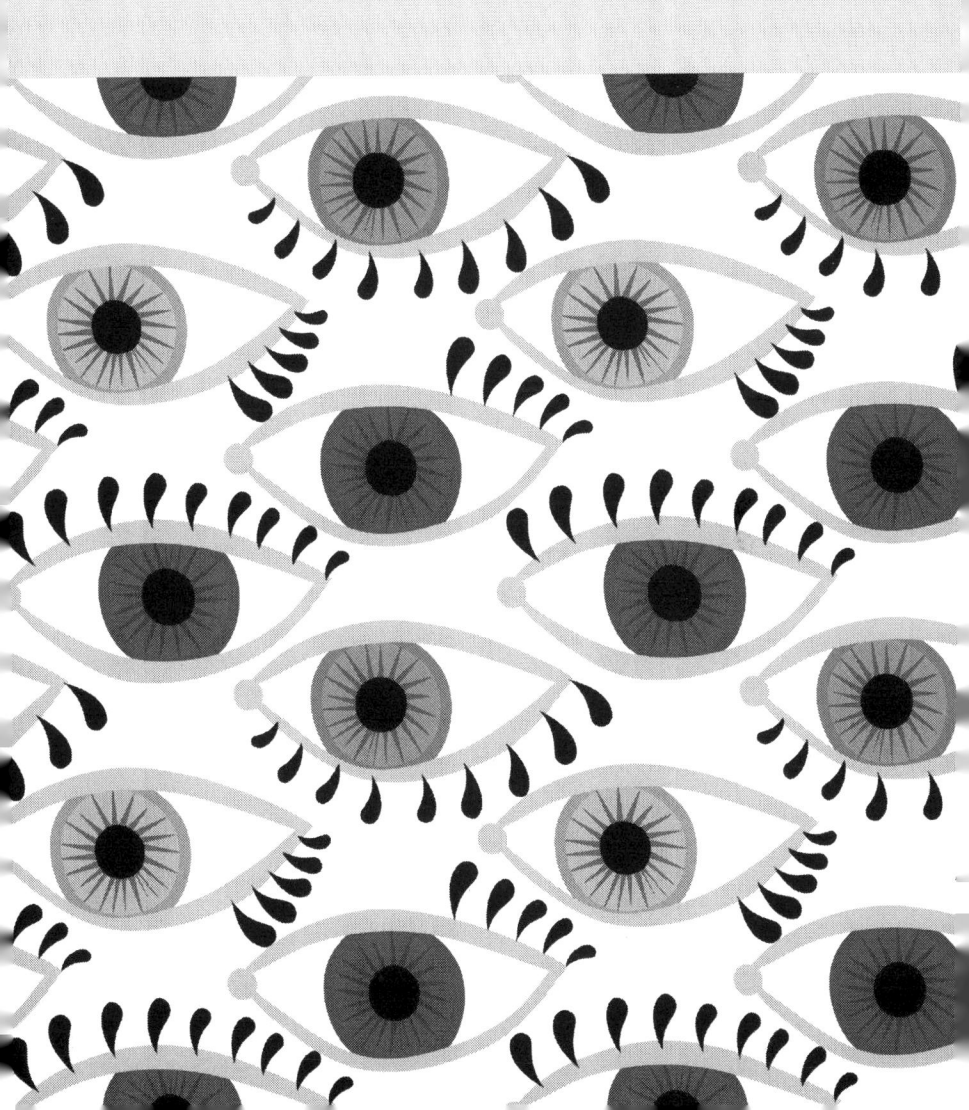

THE UGLY

10

DIABETES EYE COMPLICATIONS

Both Type 1 and Type 2 *diabetes mellitus* (DM)—diseases involving high blood sugar or glucose—can adversely contribute to a variety of "ugly" cataract surgery complications. DM can lead to disease in many tissues in the eye structure. Cataracts are one of the major causes of blindness in diabetic patients. And diabetics frequently need cataract surgery at an earlier age than non-diabetics.

According to the International Diabetes Foundation, the prevalence of DM is rapidly increasing, with an estimated total of 439 million DM patients worldwide by 2030. DM patients are reported to be at least five times more likely to develop cataracts than people without DM.

Although cataract surgery is a generally safe procedure for diabetic patients, they still are at an elevated risk of vision-impairment complications, including *diabetic retinopathy, macular edema,* and *posterior capsular opacification*. Nonetheless, just because you have diabetes does not mean that you will have any or all these conditions. Studies suggest that diabetic patients have enjoyed improved results when phacoemulsification is used during surgery. (Please see Chapter 5 for an explanation of phacoemulsification.)

Diabetic Retinopathy

Diabetic retinopathy (DR) is one of the most common and serious conditions regarding the success of cataract surgery. Diabetic retinopathy occurs when there is cumulative damage to tiny blood vessels in the retina that are caused by high blood sugar levels.

The two forms of diabetic retinopathy are called non-proliferative and proliferative. *Non-proliferative retinopathy*, the more common form, occurs when the capillaries in the back of the eye hemorrhage and leak fluid onto the retina. Damage from non-proliferative retinopathy can also cause blood spots and yellow fatty deposits on the retina. Non-proliferative retinopathy usually requires treatment when the leaking fluid causes the macula to swell to the point of causing blurry central vision.

Cataract surgery usually is successful on an eye that has diabetic non-proliferative retinopathy if the macula is not swollen or leaking. If there is a macula issue, you most likely would need to see a retina specialist for laser treatment before considering cataract surgery.

The more serious form of DR is called *proliferative retinopathy*. This condition is so progressive that the blood vessels become damaged to the point that they close completely, preventing blood to flow through the retina. When this happens, nature responds by having the retina develop its own capillaries through a process called *neovascularization*. The newly grown blood vessels however are generally so weak that they tend to leak. This leakage can cause additional damage that can lend itself to severe central and peripheral vision loss.

Cataract surgery can be iffy on an eye that suffers from proliferative retinopathy. Your eye surgeon (and/or ophthalmologist), retina specialist, and primary care physician should confer on whether to proceed or not with cataract surgery.

Keep in mind that cataract surgery cannot reverse vision impairment caused by proliferative retinopathy. This serious condition is a reminder why it is imperative to get regular eye exams, with the intent to catch progressive diseases such as diabetic retinopathy.

Macular Edema

The development of macular edema (ME) or swelling, a frequent cause of vision deterioration after surgery, is not uncommon among the general population. Fortunately, ME usually is treatable with anti-inflammatory eye drop medications.

Diabetic patients with pre-existing retinopathy, however, have an increased risk of ME after cataract surgery, according to a 2019 study published in the *World Journal of Diabetes*. In addition, this risk is proportional to the increased severity of DR. Furthermore, after successful cataract surgery, researchers found an increased retinal thickness in the eyes of diabetic patients without DR.

Posterior Capsular Opacification

Posterior capsular opacification (PCO) is one of the most common causes of impaired vision in diabetic patients. A long-term complication of cataract surgery that also can affect non-diabetics,

PCO entails scar tissue of the membrane that previously surrounded the natural lens that results in blurry vision. "Proliferation of lens epithelial cells and the degree of postoperative inflammation are associated with the development of PCO," stated the authors of a May 2019 European review entitled, "Diabetes and Phacoemulsification Cataract Surgery: Difficulties, Risks and Potential Complications", published in the *Journal of Clinical Medicine*.

PCO, also referred to as a secondary cataract or membrane, happens to about 20 to 25 percent of all cataract patients. Fortunately, a painless, 30-second procedure called *YAG laser capsulotomy* (please refer to the Glossary) can be performed on a small YAG laser machine (looks like a slit lamp) in the ophthalmologist's office. YAG laser treatment is usually successful and effective.

Let's look at a condition with which you might not be familiar with: dysphotopsia.

11

DYSPHOTOPSIA

Dysphotopsia is a word that you hope no one in your eye doctor's office mentions to you. It really means having an unwanted image in your eye. Unfortunately, dysphotopsia can occur after "perfect" cataract surgery. This ugly disorder, one of the more frequent patient complaints after successful cataract surgery (about 20 percent of cataract patients), is usually characterized as "positive" or "negative."

Positive Dyphotopsia

Positive dysphotopsia happens when a cataract patient notices unwanted light—including a starburst, halo, streak, flicker—in the operated eye. The primary cause of positive dysphotopsia is wearing square-edged, acrylic IOLs. The bad news is that most IOLs have square edges! (Square-edge IOLs have been popular since the mid-1990s because they may minimize the development of scar tissue around the IOL.) Many of these modern-era IOLs are composed of acrylic and offer higher surface reflectivity.

Keeping these facts in mind, you can discuss potential issues with your ophthalmologist *before* selecting your IOL. In other words, ask if you can consider an IOL made with silicone or copolymer rather than acrylic especially if the prescription of the IOL is a higher index of refraction.

Another post-surgery option is to replace your IOL with an IOL that has a lower index of refraction and less surface reflectivity. The ugly aspect of this alternative is undergoing cataract surgery on the same eye again.

Negative Dysphotopsia

Negative dysphotopsia occurs when a cataract patient notices a black line, figure, or crescent on the periphery of one's vision. Like positive dysphotopsia, this negative type of dysphotopsia only happens after "perfect" cataract surgery. Unfortunately, little has been accomplished in the ophthalmology world to resolve this ugly issue because its cause is controversial.

"The exact cause of these negative dysphotopsias is elusive. There's not a lab test you can get to prove what's causing them. And there is no tried-and-true, slam-dunk treatment that will work in every patient," stated Jonathan M. Davidorf, MD, who teaches ophthalmology at the University of California, Los Angeles (UCLA).

Nonetheless, a couple preventive options might be useful. One possibility is for the eye surgeon to orient the IOL's optic-haptic (handle-like, side structures that hold the IOL in place) junctions at the 3 and 9 o'clock positions in the capsular bag. By doing this, additional rays of light will scatter into the area that might otherwise be a shadow.

Another option is to apply lessons learned from the outcome of the first-eye surgery. In other words, if the right eye demonstrates negative dysphotopsia, the surgeon should consider implanting an IOL that is non-acrylic and offers a lower refractive index in the left eye.

Surgical approaches are also possibilities to treat negative dysphotopsia. For example, if non-surgical options fail, the IOL that is apparently causing negative dysphotopsia can be replaced with an IOL that has a larger optic. Steven I. Rosenfeld, MD, an eye surgeon in Delray Beach, California, offered, "…there's some clinical evidence that IOLs with smaller optics are more inclined to have dysphotopsias. So, I'm less inclined to leave a 5-mm optic in the eye. In contrast, if a patient has a lens optic of 6 mm or greater, I'm more inclined to leave that lens in place and try something like reverse optic capture."

Several ophthalmologists from the David Geffen School of Medicine-UCLA, Stein Eye Institute in Los Angeles, California evaluated preventative and curative surgical strategies for negative dysphotopsia. Their conclusion is called a *reverse optic capture*. Published in a January 2018 issue of *the Journal of Cataract & Refractive Surgery*, their study concluded that "negative dysphotopsia was reduced, eliminated, or prevented when the IOL optic overlaid the anterior capsulotomy rather than when the capsule edge overlaid the optic."

The next chapter addresses the serious disorder called macular degeneration.

12

MACULAR DEGENENERATION

"Macular degeneration" comprises two words that you do not want to hear an eye doctor say to you. Yet statistics indicate this serious eye condition is becoming more common as populations age.

At least sixteen million persons in the United States have been diagnosed with age-related macular degeneration. In the year 2020, public health officials estimated that the number of people with macular degeneration will reach 196 million globally.

Risk factors of macular degeneration include smoking, obesity, high blood pressure, and family history of *age-related macular degeneration* (AMD).

In fact, AMD is quite prevalent in Caucasian males aged 80 or older.

The macula is a circular centralized area of the retina; it produces highly detailed central vision. Degeneration of the macula can make cataract surgery more complex.

However, researchers from the prestigious Wills Eye Hospital in Philadelphia, Pennsylvania reviewed evidence that AMD subjects enjoyed "improved visual acuity, absence of significant disease progression, and improved quality of life" by undergoing cataract surgery. Their study was published in a 2017 issue of the journal *Current Opinion in Ophthalmology*.

Age-Related Macular Degeneration

As we age, the macula muscle can deteriorate and damage the light-sensitive macular cells. AMD adversely affects your ability to read, drive, or perform close-up tasks. Unfortunately, there is no cure for this disease. But prescribed eye drops and injections are known to slow the pace of AMD. As with all "bad" and "ugly" conditions, contact your eye specialist as soon as possible to mitigate the possible worsening of the condition.

Dry Macular Degeneration

Dry macular degeneration is the least serious form of the three types. Dry macular degeneration happens when the macular cells slowly deteriorate, causing a gradual loss of vision. A tip-off to dry macular degeneration is seeing straight lines that appear crooked or wavy. Unfortunately, there is no effective treatment for this type of macular degeneration. Maintaining excellent nutrition however may slow the progression of this disease. (Please refer to the bonus chapter on Eye Nutrition near the end of this book for nutritional information that may help to slow the deterioration of the macula).

Wet Macular Degeneration

Wet macular degeneration is more serious than the "dry" version. Wet macular degeneration is when abnormal blood vessels develop under the macula. These blood vessels leak fluid that damage the macular tissues and cause not only crooked lines but other eye problems including blurriness. If you have these symptoms, run, don't walk to your ophthalmologist for treatment to save what vision remains in the macula. Treatment for wet macular degeneration includes injections to inhibit abnormal blood vessel growth and laser therapy to stop the leakage of fluid.

The end of this chapter leads us to the final "ugly" chapter that covers a wide range of eye conditions that hopefully you will never encounter after cataract surgery.

13

POST-SURGERY COMPLICATIONS

"Ugly" cataract-related complications are untoward, but they do happen. For example, I surmise that my mother probably endured corneal edema during her first eye cataract surgery. She was too exhausted as a caregiver to family members to pursue complex surgeries. Decades later, she suffers daily with corneal swelling.

Most of the incidents addressed in this chapter are due to intraoperative mistakes that can be easily avoided. Once again, I cannot over-emphasize the need to enlist an eye surgeon who holds an impeccible success rate as a "cataract surgeon."

Corneal Edema

After cataract surgery, the cornea—the clear window in front of the eye—can gather fluid that causes swelling. Most swelling is normal and may last a few days.

It is possible, though, to experience persistent corneal swelling, blurred vision, and eye pain. An ugly solution to unrelenting corneal swelling is to undergo a corneal graft procedure where the damaged cornea is removed and replaced by donor tissue.

Indian researchers conclude in a study, published in December 2017, that corneal edema is an avoidable complication. They state that "careful preoperative workup, intraoperative precautions and vigilant postoperative care" are necessary for successful surgery.

Dislocated IOL

A dislocated intraocular lens (IOL) should not happen but it does. Remember that an IOL is designed to be held securely in the posterior chamber but sometimes it slips.

A variety of reasons for this rare complication include: 1) weakness of the fibers (zonules) that hold the chamber membrane in place, 2) pseudoexfoliation (please see the Pseuodoexfoliation section of this chapter), 3) a genetic disorder called Marfan's syndrome, and 4) another genetic condition called *homocystinuria* that involves misprocessing amino acids.

If a dislocated IOL is causing issues such as halos, faded or double vision, shimmering images, your eye surgeon may need to remove and reposition the lens. Hopefully, an IOL, although dislocated, will remain positioned centrally and not distort your vision.

Endophthalmitis

While eye infection from cataract surgery is rare, it can lead to damage of the inner eye lid or a condition called endophthalmitis. Symptoms of endophthalmitis include reddish and swollen eyes, severe pain, and possibly loss of vision. Diligent application of antibiotic eye drops before, during, and after surgery should obviate the likelihood of endophthalmitis.

Posterior Capsule Rupture

An example of a truly ugly event is when the transparent membrane of the posterior capsular bag, which holds the lens (natural or IOL), ruptures.

Unfortunately, a rupture of this type cannot be repaired. In this case, the eye surgeon would need to perform a more complicated procedure: remove the vitreous gel from the center of the eyeball and implant the IOL about a millimeter in front of the area where it normally is placed. This solution is not ideal but ultimately may offer a viable result.

Pseudoexfoliation

Pseuodoexfoliation (PEX) is a major risk factor for complications during cataract surgery. In addition, PEX is the most prevalent cause of secondary glaucoma, which you know occurs after cataract surgery.

This complex and aging-related disorder is often referred to as "eye dandruff." Microscopic white or grey protein fibers, resembling skin dandruff flakes, populate the front surface of the lens, iris, and pupil as well as the eye drainage system called the trabecular meshwork.

You may recall that a thin, pocket-like structure or transparent capsular bag houses the natural lens or IOL. Tiny ligaments called *zonules* support the lens in its capsular bag behind the iris.

However, eye injuries, prior eye surgeries, and aging can stretch or weaken the zonules, exacerbating cataract surgery because the weak capsular bag is challenged to house an IOL. One treatment during cataract surgery is to place a microscopic, plastic stabilization ring into the capsular bag.

Pseudoexfoliation is more common in older Caucasian persons of Northern European, Scandinavian, and/or Russian heritage. The disorder is also more prevalent in females than males. In addition, prematurely born children are susceptible to an eye condition called *retinopathy of prematurity*, which can cause weak ligaments that will later lend themselves to PEX.

Researchers also discovered an association between PEX and genetic variants in a gene called *LOX1*. The LOX1 gene regulates *elastin*, a protein that facilitates connective tissue to return to its original position when touched or prodded. When the LOX1 gene variant is expressed, it may exacerbate the effectiveness of the elastins, causing potential surgical implications.

Posterior Vitreous Detachment

Posterior vitreous detachment (PVD) sounds bad, and it can be. PVD can happen without cataract surgery to patients who have high myopia (extreme nearsightedness).

In essence, PVD takes place as a chain reaction: as vitreous fluid in our eyes thins with age and/or cataract surgery, the posterior, or back, part of the gel shrinks and tugs at retinal fibers in one spot on the retina.

But PVD also can occur months after a successful cataract operation. As the new IOL is thinner than the natural lens it replaced, extraneous space from the gap in the capsular bag facilitates the vitreous fluid pulling on retinal fibers.

Visual clues for PVD include seeing images such as cob-web floaters and looking through a steamed window. See a retinal ophthalmologist soonest if you notice these indicators.

Retinal Detachment

Speaking about retinal issues, a serious potential issue after cataract surgery is when the retina detaches from the inner eye wall, called *retinal detachment*. We already talked about PVD, which could lead to actual detachment of the retina.

Seeing flashing stars or light is a tell-tale sign of retinal detachment. If this happens to one or both eyes, run, don't walk, to your eye doctor. Call this person immediately! Prompt attention to reattaching the blood vessels that nourish the eye back to the retinal wall should save your eye and its vision. Remember, retinal detachment, a possible side effect of cataract surgery, can lead to blindness if not treated in a highly timely fashion.

Suprachoroidal Hemorrhage

"*Suprachoroidal hemorrhage* (SCH) is a rare but potentially devastating complication in intraocular surgery," stated Singaporean researchers in the May 2018 issue of *EyeNet Magazine*. They conceded however that the incidence of SCH during cataract surgery has decreased over the past twenty-five years, owing to improved surgical techniques and equipment.

SCH occurs when blood accumulates within the space between the choroid and the sclera. The choroid is a layer of vascular layer of connective tissue. The sclera simply is the "white of the eye."

Risk factors for the increase SCH include advanced age, hypertension (high blood pressure), peripheral vascular disease, and blood thinners as well as other cardiovascular drugs. In addition, eye conditions that heighten the possibility of having an SCH include high myopia (nearsightedness), glaucoma, elevated preoperative IOP, and a previous intraocular surgery.

This chapter concludes the "ugly" part of *The Eyes Have It*. Please read on for a brief wrap-up and a bonus chapter about eye nutrition.

CONCLUDING THOUGHTS

Cataract surgery enjoys a high success rate. My cataract surgeries fortunately went well. Having successful cataract surgery is a gift of better eyesight. That's "The Good."

Pre-existing conditions however can complicate undergoing cataract operations. That's "The Bad." These include complicated eyes, glaucoma, and LASIK. "The Bad" also addresses the potential issue of wearing eyeglasses.

Unfortunately, nasty issues can happen due to cataract surgery. That's "The Ugly." While I hesitated to write about "The Ugly," I felt it was necessary to inform you, the reader, about what can go wrong. About ten percent of cataract operations do not go well. Therefore, it is imperative that you have full confidence in your eye surgeon. I cannot overemphasize this!

An excellent ophthalmologist, who specializes in cataract surgery, will assist you in selecting the best intraocular lens and type of cataract surgery for you. Receiving the best lens implant and type of surgery is paramount to your successful operation.

I sincerely hope you have found this book to be helpful. Whether you are contemplating cataract surgery, have undergone it, or want to assist a friend or loved one with the process and the pitfalls, *The Eyes Have It* should be useful.

Remember, I was "scared to death" of undergoing cataract surgery, and I survived with a smile, energy, and enthusiasm to share my experiences and knowledge in this book. Best wishes!

~ Susan Rex Ryan

P.S. If you found the information in this book useful, please consider posting a brief review on Amazon. Thank you so much.

BONUS CHAPTER: EYE NUTRITION

"Eat your carrots," my mother said insistently. "Eat your carrots, they are good for your eyes!"

This six-year-old defiantly pouted and pushed the disc-shaped, buttered carrots around on her plate.

Did I end up eating those carrots? No, but I never forgot the connection between carrots and healthy eyes. Why are carrots good for your eyes? You will find out in this chapter.

Good nutrition, primarily from your diet, plays an important role in maintaining healthy eyes and may increase your chances that you will enjoy successful cataract surgery. There is no credible evidence however that your diet can prevent the development of cataracts.

Let's look at a brief discussion about eye nutrition.

Vitamin A

Vitamin A (fat-soluble) and beta carotene are involved in the metabolism, growth, and differentiation of the outer-most surface of the cornea. Carrots indeed are bountiful in beta carotene, a carotenoid pigment that is an important precursor to vitamin A and responsible for carrots' orange coloring. Beta carotene is also found in lots of other vegetables and fruits.

In the Western world, vitamin A deficiency is rare. But in developing countries low vitamin A levels comprise one of the primary causes of preventable blindness.

Since vitamin A supplementation is usually unnecessary in developed countries, avoid taking vitamin A pills. In fact, a note of caution: when cod liver oil (rich in vitamin A) or retinol supplements containing retinyl acetate and retinyl palmitate are taken, vitamin A toxicity may occur. Excess vitamin A in the body may cause havoc because it denies other vitamins, including vitamin D3, from influencing genetic activity.

Vitamin D3

Speaking of fat-soluble nutrients, vitamin D3 plays an important role in eye health. Virtually every cell in the eye contains a vitamin D3 receptor. When they receive adequate vitamin D3, these receptors participate in regulating immune actions, cellular proliferation, differentiation, apoptosis, and genetic activity, which in turn enhance corneal (as well as other parts of the eye) functions.

Italian researchers found that vitamin D3 supplementation significantly improved dry eye disease symptoms. The science was published in the March 2020 issue of the journal *Nutrients*. Another 2020 study, reported in the journal *Contact Lens and Anterior Eye*," concludes that "vitamin D plays an important role in human eye health."

Western diets contain little vitamin D3. Therefore, D3 supplementation is the most effective way to raise your serum vitamin D3 level. A safe daily dose of 10,000 vitamin D3 international units along with 200 mcg of vitamin K2 MK-7 <u>for people without kidney or liver disease</u> should help elevate your serum D3 level to an optimal 100 ng/mL (250 nmol/L).

The eye is only one organ in the human body that requires lots of vitamin D3 to function properly. Our entire body needs vitamin D3. For additional information on vitamin D3 and its amazing health benefits, check out the *Defend Your Life* vitamin D3 books.

Lutein and Zeaxanthin

When I think of specific nutrients for the eyes, I think of lutein and its partner zeaxanthin. Only these two carotenoids, of which there are about 600 in nature, accumulate in high amounts in the macula. These carotenoids may be effective in filtering harmful, high-energy blue light, offering anti-inflammatory properties, and maintaining healthy cells in the eye.

Lutein and zeaxanthin supplements are readily available online or in retail stores. I have been taking a 20-mg soft gel capsule containing these special carotenoids for years; my ophthalmologist has consistently remarked about the positive health of my eyes. Since lutein and zeaxanthin have a half-life of ten days, you only need to take one supplement every ten days.

Vitamin C

Water-soluble vitamin C, plentiful in citrus fruits, can enhance the absorption of lutein in the eye. The good news here is that vitamin C supplements may slow the progression of age-related macular degeneration (AMD). Researchers concluded that the second National Eye Institute's Age-Related Eye Disease Study (AREDS2) suggests that taking certain vitamins including vitamin C may slow

the progression of AMD. They cautioned however that vitamins cannot prevent the onset of AMD.
The AREDS2 researchers recommended taking at least 500 mg of vitamin C a day. Vitamin C tablets are widely commercially available.

Vitamin E

Fat-soluble vitamin E is resplendent in antioxidants, which may protect the eyes from free radicals that could delay the development of AMD. Vitamin E can be found in green vegetables, nuts, and fortified foods. Vitamin E may lower the odds of developing AMD and cataracts but there is insufficient evidence to indicate that taking vitamin E supplements will halt the progress of cataracts and AMD.

It is better to acquire vitamin E from your diet. However, recommended supplement dosing is no more than 50 mg daily.

Selenium

The trace mineral selenium acts as an antioxidant. For eye health, selenium's primary function is to promote the absorption of vitamin E. The ARENDS study suggested that adequate selenium in the body may help prevent diabetic retinopathy (see Chapter 10). Selenium also may slow the progression of eye issues related to Grave's disease, an autoimmune disorder affecting the thyroid.

The best natural source of selenium is a Brazil nut. Yes, that is singular word, one Brazil nut provides the daily recommended allowance of 55 mcg daily. In my opinion, it is best to not supplement with selenium as a miniscule amount goes a long way. Excess selenium may lead to toxicity, symptoms of which include bad breath, nausea, diarrhea, skin rashes, and irritability.

Zinc

The trace mineral zinc works with vitamin A in the retina to produce melanin, a protective pigment in the eyes. Zinc is highly concentrated in the eye, primarily in the retina and choroid.

Zinc is commonly found in red meats, shellfish, beans, poultry, and nuts. Zinc deficiency is rare; therefore, most people do not need to supplement with it. If you do choose to supplement with zinc, take no more than 50 mg per day.

Eye Nutrition: Conclusion

As with any organ in our body, our eyes need a certain amount and various types of nutrition.

Most healthy diets include the vitamins and minerals for our eyes to function well.

The only supplements that I take for my eyes are a lutein (20-mg) and 2-mg zeaxanthin soft gel capsule as well as a combination of vitamins D3 (10,000 iu) and 200-mcg K2 MK-7 soft gel capsules. When shopping for supplements, I always read the ingredients labels carefully and select the one(s) with the least amount of ingredients as some could be unhelpful fillers.

Prior to taking over-the-counter supplements, find out what is best for you and your eye health. The decision about your eye nutrition should be done in concert with your eye doctor's recommendations.

INDEX

A
alpha-crystallins 7
astigmatism 18

C
Cambodia 53
capsular bag 56
carotenoid 92
choroid 87
complicated eyes 55
congenital 8
cornea 18
corneal edema 82
cortical cataracts 8

D
diabetes mellitus 67
diabetic retinopathy 68
diopters 20
dry eye 62
dry macular degeneration 79
dysphotopsia 71

E
edema 70

endophthalmitis 64, 83
extracapsular cataract extraction 37
eyeglasses 2

F
femtosecond (FS) laser 19, 20, 37
floaters 62

G
glaucoma 57
gritty sensation 63

H
halo 8, 73

I
intraocular lens (IOL) 18
intraocular pressure (IOP) 57
iris 56

L
LASIK 24, 59

limbal relaxing incision 20, 24
LOX1 85
lutein 94

M
macula 69
macular degeneration 77
macular edema 68
mini-mono 26
mini-mono vision 19
monofocal intraocular lens (IOL) 19, 37
monovision 26
multifocal IOL 20, 27
multifocal lens 19
myopia 85

N
negative dysphotopsia 74
neovascularization 69
non-proliferative retinopathy 68
NSAID 22
nuclear cataract 8

O
ophthalmic viscoelastic devices (OVDs) 63
ophthalmologist 6
optical nerve 57
optician 53

P
phacoemulsification 37
pilocarpine 56
positive dysphotopsia 73
posterior capsular opacification 68
posterior capsule rupture 83
posterior vitreous detachment 85
prednisone 40
presbyopia 18, 50
proliferative retinopathy 69
pseudoexfoliation 57
pupil 56

R
refractive 24
retina 7
retinal detachment 86
Ridley, Harold, M.D. 25

S
sclera 87
secondary glaucoma 64
selenium 95
slit lamp 43
speculum 36
stitch 43
subcapsular cataracts 8
suprachoroidal hemorrhage 62

T

tonometry 57
toric lens 27
trabelculectomy 57
traumatic cataracts 9

V

vitamin A 92
vitamin C 94
vitamin D3 92
vitamin E 95
vitrectomy 60

W

wet macular degeneration 79

Y

YAG 71

Z

zeaxanthin 94
zinc 96
zonules 56

GLOSSARY

Alpha-crystallins: protective proteins in the eye. When these proteins clump together in the natural eye lens, a cataract can form.

Astigmatism: non-spherical shape of the cornea that can cause blurring at all distances.

Capsular bag: holds the eye lens. The bag is suspended by zonules, thousands of microscopic fibers.

Carotenoids: a class of plant chemicals that contains primarily orange, yellow, and red fat-soluble pigments.

Cataract: the clouding of the natural eye lens that can cause visual impairment and blindness. Types of cataracts include nuclear, cortical, subcapsular, congenital, and traumatic.

Choroid: a vascular layer of the eye, containing connective tissues, that lies between the retina and the sclera.

Complicated eye: a term used to characterize an eye that has features that can complicate cataract surgery. An example of a complicated eye is small pupils.

Congenital cataract: when a baby is born with, or develops, a cataract.

Cornea: the clear window in front of the eye.

Corneal edema: post-surgery complication with the cornea gathering fluid that causes swelling.

Cortical cataract: the type of cataract that forms along the edge of the lens.

Diabetic retinopathy: a common but serious condition, caused by high blood pressure in diabetics, that occurs when there is cumulative damage to tiny blood vessels in the retina.

Diopter: a unit of measurement used to correct focusing power that a lens requires.

Dry eye: a common condition after cataract surgery. Treatment usually comprises lubricating the eyes with quality artificial tears.

Dysphotopsia: an "ugly" post-surgery eye disorder where an unwanted image appears in the implanted lens. Also see "Positive Dysphotopsia" and "Negative Dysphotopsia."

Edema: swelling.

Endophthalmitis: a rare condition after cataract surgery that involves damage to the inner eye lid.

Extracapsular cataract extraction: removal of the faulty natural lens (cataract).

Femtosecond laser: an FS laser machine that assists the surgeon with incisions in the eye.

Floaters: clumps of vitreous gel in the central eye cavity. Can be common before and after cataract surgery.

Glaucoma: a serious eye disease that gradually impairs peripheral vision.

Halo effect: the perception of seeing a round "halo" surrounding lights. Can be either pre- or post-surgery, depending on the situation.

Intraocular lens (IOL): an artificial lens that is implanted after cataract removal.

Intraocular pressure (IOP): built up fluid in the eye that causes IOP. If the IOP continues to increase, the pressure from the fluid can cause gradual damage to the optical nerve.
Iris: the colored part of the eye.
LASIK: stands for *"laser-assisted in situ keratomileusis."* LASIK, a type of refractive surgery, is performed by an ophthalmologist who uses a laser to reshape the cornea to improve visual acuity.
Lens: a transparent intraocular tissue that is located behind the pupil. The lens helps bring rays of light to a focus on the retina.
Limbal relaxing incision: an incision made by an FS laser machine to treat mild astigmatism.
LOX1: the gene that regulates elastin, a protein that helps connective tissue to return to its original position when touched or prodded. If the LOX1 gene is turned on, it may adversely affect the elastins. The LOX1 gene is associated with eye dandruff or pseudoexfoliation.
Lutein: a carotenoid that accumulates in the macula. A lutein nutritional supplement usually includes zeaxanthin, another carotenoid.
Macula: the functional center of the retina.
Macular degeneration: an incurable eye disease that is commonly age-related.
Macular edema: clear fluid that collects in the macula, impairing central vision.
Mini mono vision: also referred to as blended monovision. "Mini mono" encompasses one near-vision IOL in one eye and one IOL with far-vision in the other eye.

Monofocal IOL: the most common type of IOL; provides either near or distance vision.

Multifocal IOL: a newer-generation IOL that provides a visual range for near, intermediate, and far visions. This type of IOL works similarly to progressive lenses in eyeglasses.

Myopia: nearsightedness.

Neovascularization: a process that happens in response to proliferative retinopathy. The retina develops its own capillaries through this process. However, the capillaries are usually weak and tend to bleed, which could cause severe damage.

Non-proliferative diabetic retinopathy: the more common form of diabetic retinopathy.

NSAID: non-steroidal anti-inflammatory drug. Ibuprofen is a common NSAID.

Nuclear cataract: the most common type of age-related cataracts. Hazy vision is mainly in the center of the lens.

Ophthalmologist: a medical or osteopathic doctor who specializes in eye and vision care. An ophthalmologist typically completes at least twelve years of training and education and is licensed to practice medicine and surgery. An ophthalmologist performs cataract surgery.

Optic nerve: located in the back of the eye, an optic nerve transfers, via electrical impulses, visual information from the retina to visual centers in the eye.

Optician: a technician who is trained to design, verify, and fit eyeglass lenses and frames, and contact lenses to correct eyesight. Opticians are not permitted to diagnose or treat eye diseases.

Optometrist: a healthcare professional who provides vision services. An optometrist is not a medical doctor but must be licensed as a Doctor of Optometry (OD). An optician's range of eye care varies from state to state.

Phacoemulsification: a newer technique for the extraction procedure during cataract surgery.

Posterior capsular opacification (PCO): one of the most common causes of impaired vision in diabetic patients. Posterior capsule: the back of the capsule that holds the lens.

Posterior capsule rupture: A highly serious condition when the transparent membrane of the posterior capsule bag ruptures.

Posterior chamber IOL: the back area of an intraocular lens.

Posterior vitreous detachment: a serious retinal condition that can occur pre- or post-surgery.

Prednisone: a type of prescription steroid medication.

Presbyopia: a common eye condition that occurs when flexible muscles that hold the natural lens begin to stiffen with age. Cataract surgery literally disconnects those muscles from the natural lens. In other words, cataract surgery patients will become presybyopic unless they purchase a presbyopia correcting IOL.

Proliferative diabetic retinopathy: a progressive disease in diabetics when the blood vessels become damaged, preventing blood flow to the retina. This condition leads to neovascularization (defined in this glossary).

Pseudoexfoliation: also known as "eye dandruff."

Pupil: the natural window into the eye.

Refractive surgery: surgery to improve vision such as LASIK.
Retina: sitting in the back of the eye, the retina is a thin layer of tissue that enables vision.
Retinal detachment: the retina detaches from the inner eye wall.
Sclera: the white part of the eye.
Secondary glaucoma: an increase in eye pressure after cataract surgery.
Selenium: a trace mineral that acts as an antioxidant.
Slit lamp: an ophthalmic instrument that includes a microscope with a bright light and is used during an eye exam. Glaucoma test equipment is commonly mounted on the slit lamp.
Speculum: a device that holds open the eyelids during eye surgery.
Subcapsular cataract: a cataract that develops rapidly and can begin at the front or the back of the lens.
Suprachoroidal hemorrhage: a rare condition that occurs when blood accumulates within the space between the choroid and sclera.
Tonometry: testing to measure eye pressure.
Toric IOL: toric lenses are designed fix or decrease pronounced astigmatism.
Traumatic cataract: a cataract that forms from an eye injury.
Vitrectomy: involves outpatient surgery to treat issues with the retina and vitreous, a gel-like substance that fills about two-thirds of the eyes. which can be removed during a vitrectomy.
Wet macular degeneration: a serious condition when abnormal blood vessels develop under the macula.

YAG: scientific name is "Nnd: yag neodymium: Yttrium – Aluminum Garnet; easier to call the laser treatment "YAG." An outpatient procedure that removes scar tissue developed from cataract surgery.

Zeaxanthin: a carotenoid that works in tandem with lutein to maintain healthy cells in the eye.

Zonules: microscopic ligaments that support the lens and capsular bag.

BIBLIOGRAPHY

Absher, Kenneth J. "How to Improve Your Odds of Successful Cataract Surgery." *Life Extension*. 2015 Nov; 69-71.

Askari, G et al. "Association between vitamin D and dry eye disease: A systematic review and meta-analysis of observational studies." *Contact Lens and Anterior Eye*. 2020 Mar 10. Pii:S1367-9484(20)30039-4.

Buscemi, Silvio et al. "The Effect of Lutein on Eye and Extra-Eye Health." *Nutrients*. 2018 Sep 18;10(9) pii:E1321.

Chang, David F. "The Continuing Evolution of Cataract Surgery." *Asia-Pacific Journal of Ophthalmology*. 2017 July;6(4):308.

Chang, David F. and Lee, Bryan S. *Cataracts: A Patient's Guide to Treatment*, Slack Incorporated, 2016.

Demirci, G et al. "Dry Eye Assessment in Patients with Vitamin D Deficiency" *Eyes and Contact Lens*. 2018 Sep;44 Suppl. 1:S62-S65.

Ehmann, David S. and Ho, Allen C. "Cataract Surgery and Age-Related Macular Degeneration." *Current Opinion in Ophthalmology*. 2017 Jan;28(1):58-62.

Faloon, Patricia. "Cataract Surgery: Beware…Be Aware." *Life Extension*. 2015 Nov; 72-76.

Foo, Reuben et al. "Management of Suprachoroidal Hemorrhage." *EyeNet Magazine*, 2018 May.

Garland, Paul E., MD and Fisher, Bret L., *Cataract Surgery: A Guide to Treatment,* Addicus Books, 2015.

Gibbons, A et al. "Causes and correction of dissatisfaction after implantation of presbyopia-correcting intraocular lenses." *Journal of Clinical Ophthalmology.* 2018 Oct 11;10:1965-1970.

Gorusupudi, Aruna et al. "The Age-Related Eye Disease 2 Study: Micronutrients in the Treatment of Macular Degeneration." *Advances in Nutrition.* 2017 Jan;8(1):40-53.

Grzybowski, Andrzej et al. "Diabetes and Phacoemulsification Cataract Surgery: Difficulties, Risks and Potential Complications." *Journal of Clinical Medicine.* 2019 May 20;8(5). Pii:E716.

Holladay, Jack T. and Simpson, Michael J. "Negative Dysphotopsia: Causes and Rationale for Prevention and Treatment." *Journal of Cataract & Refractive Surgery.* 2017 Feb;43(2):263-275.

Ishrat, Saba et al. "Incidence and Pattern of Dry Eye After Cataract Surgery." *Saudi Journal of Ophthalmology.* 2019 Jan-Mar;33(1):34-40.

Kim, Jinsoo et al. "Comparison of Floaters after Cataract Surgery with Different Viselastics." *International Journal of Medical Sciences.* 2018; 15(3):223-227.

Kiziltoprak, Hasan et al. "Cataract in diabetes mellitus." *World Journal of Diabetes.* 2019 Mar 15;10(3):140-153.

Khoo, Hock Eng et al. "Nutrients for Prevention of Macular Degeneration and Eye-Related Diseases." *Antioxidants* (Basel)" 2019 Apr 2;8(4):85.

Masket, Samuel et al. "Surgical Management of Negative Dysphotopsia." *Journal of Cataract & Refractive Surgery*. 2018 Jan;44(1):6-16.

Pelligrini, Marco et al. "The Role of Nutrition and Nutritional Supplements in Ocular Surface Diseases." *Nutrients*. 2020 Mar 30;12(4):952.

Roach, Linda. "Shedding Light on Pseudophakic Dysphotopsia." *EyeNet Magazine*. 2014 December.

Rullo, J et al. "Intraocular calcidiol: Uncovering a role for vitamin D in the eye." *The Journal of Steroid Biochemistry and Molecular Biology*. 2020 Mar; 197:105536.

Sharma, Namrata et al. "Corneal edema after phacoemulsification." *Indian Journal of Ophthalmology*. 2017 Dec; 65(12):1381-1389.

Stein, Joshua D. "Serious Adverse Events After Cataract Surgery." *Current Opinion in Ophthalmology Journal*. 2012 May;23(3):23(3)219-25.

Suryawanshi, M and Alsaidi, R. "Femtosecond laser-assisted cataract surgery." *Oman Journal of Ophthalmology*. 2020 Jan-Apr;13(1):1-2.

Tekin, Kamal et al. "Monitoring and management of the patient with pseudoexfoliation syndrome: current perspectives." *Journal of Clinical Ophthalmology*. 2019 March;13:453-464.

ACKNOWLEDGMENTS

The support of my wonderful husband Dave helped me get through those long days of researching the scientific literature and writing this book. His love and care also helped me cope with the apprehension instilled in me. Dave also patiently administrated the myriad rounds of eye drops which are essential to successful recovery.

I would like to thank my ophthalmologist, his caring staff, and the surgery center in Las Vegas, Nevada who ensured that I had successful cataract surgery.

Special thanks to Cheryl Strayed, *New York Times* #1 bestselling author of *Wild*. Five years ago, I was fortunate to study writing under Cheryl's sage tutelage. Her self-confidence, writing skills, and courage inspired me to tell my story about what had been the unthinkable for me: cataract surgery.

The cover and interior design of *The Eyes Have It* are products of a superb graphic design professional named Shannon Bodie of BookWise Design in Oregon. The visual magic performed by Shannon and her team enhances the feel and content of this book.

I also would like to thank the women and men in science who have devoted themselves to improve aspects of cataract surgery. Millions of us benefit from their research.

ABOUT THE AUTHOR

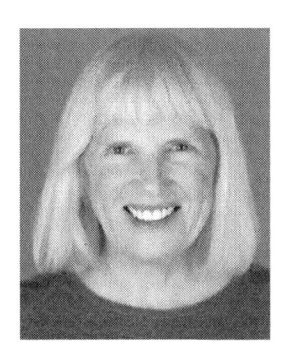

Susan "Sue" Rex Ryan was born and raised in the Philadelphia, Pennsylvania area. She earned a Bachelor of Science degree at Georgetown University. Sue also holds a Master of Science degree from the U.S. military's National War College in Washington, D.C. In addition, she has earned scores of Continuing Medical Education (CME) credits from accredited U.S. medical programs approved by, *inter alia*, The American Academy of Family Physicians.

Sue's first book entitled *Defend Your Life* discusses the many health benefits of vitamin D and has garnered global accolades as an Amazon bestseller. In addition, *Defend Your Life* won a prestigious Mom's Choice Award®, an international awards program that recognizes authors and others for their efforts in creating quality family-friendly media products.

The Eyes Have It: A Patient's Insights into Cataract Surgery is Sue's fourth health-related book. Noting a paucity of easy-to-read, patient-written books about cataract surgery, she has shared her experience as a reluctant cataract surgery patient. Although her experience was positive, Sue also explains the numerous pitfalls one may encounter from cataract surgery.

Sue and her husband Dave reside in the sunny suburbs of beautiful Las Vegas, Nevada. They enjoy traveling to visit family and friends, as well as experiencing life in far-flung locations including Sri Lanka, Easter Island, and French Polynesia.

Follow Sue's commentary on Twitter @ **vitD3Sue**. She welcomes your visit to her website **smilinsuepubs.com** that is replete with her blog articles about health topics.

Made in the USA
Columbia, SC
02 May 2025